I0464194

It's Time
To See
The
DOCTOR

Second Edition

DR . K. Murugesan M.B.B.S.,

It's Time To See The DOCTOR

ISBN: **1500872490**
ISBN-13: **978-1500872496**

DEDICATION

I Dedicate this book to my Teachers in Government high school,
VELLANKOIL , Tamil Nadu and KAMBAN KALVI NILAIYAM
Matriculation H r .Sec . School correspondent MR .P.P.KALIANNAN,
GOBICHETTIPALAYAM and MR .GURUSAMY ,Teacher,
GOBICHETTIPALAYAM and my School friends in VELLANKOIL
and my friend Jaya Kumar in London.

It's Time To See The DOCTOR

It's Time To See The DOCTOR

CONTENTS

It's Time To See The DOCTOR

ACKNOWLEDGMENTS

This book is an useful reference for general people to know when to consult a doctor and at what situations you should not miss to consult a doctor. This book illustrates common clinical complaints that needs to be consulted with the doctors. By going through this book you would consult the doctor at an early point of disease onset so that doctors would be able to give you appropriate treatment for diseases.

SUMIEYA ,CHENNAI

It's Time To See The DOCTOR

1 FEVER

Fever is a manifestation of body's defense against infection inside the body , we must consult a general physician immediately and follow his advice. You must consult the doctor as soon as possible. Fever has many causes like infection ,auto immune diseases, chronic infections, and malignancy it is very difficult for an ordinary man to tell the causes. so you must consult the doctor and he/she in his/her professional ability would be able to find out and give proper treatment .So do not Self-Medicate yourself by buying tablets of your choice in the medical shop.

If you have any of these complaints see the doctor immediately :

-High grade fever

-Fever with chills and rigors

-Fever with headache

-Fever with vomiting

-Fever with abdomen pain

-Fever with generalized body pain

-Fever with joint pain

-Fever with loose stools

-Fever with seizures

-Fever with altered mental status

-Fever with neck stiffness

-Fever with muscle pain

-Fever with puffiness of face

-Fever with swelling of joints

-Fever with blisters in the body

-Fever with rashes in the body

-Fever with bloody urine

-Fever with cough

-Fever with breathing difficulty

-Fever with blurring of vision

-Fever with cough and sputum mixed with blood

-Fever with chest pain

-Fever with palpitation

-Fever with night sweat

-Fever with lymph node enlargement

-Fever with neck swelling

-Fever with swelling in the axilla

-Fever with multiple skin excoriation in the body

It's Time To See The DOCTOR

-Fever with swelling of digits and toes

-Fever with peeling of skin in fingers and toes

-Fever with sore throat

-Fever with sore throat and inability to speak and drooling of saliva

-Fever with redness of tongue

-Fever with redness of throat

-Fever with swelling of cheeks

-Fever with reddening of eyes

-Fever with running nose

-Fever with barking cough

-Fever with high pitched cry in children

-Fever with wheezing

-Fever with Ear discharge

-Fever with ear pain

-Fever with giddiness

-Fever with unable to walk

-Fever with giddiness while standing

-Fever with wounds in the penis and vagina

-Fever with discharge in penis and vagina

-Fever with throat pain and followed by blood stained urine within one month

-Fever with dark yellow discoloration of urine

-Fever with dark yellow discoloration of eyes

-Fever occurring in the night times

-Fever with loss of weight

-Fever with loss of appetite

-Fever with generalized body swelling

-Fever with frequent urination

-Fever with pain during urination

-Fever with inability to pass urine

-Fever with lower abdomen pain

-Fever with groin pain

-Fever with swelling in scrotum

-Fever with swelling in groin area

-Fever with painful ulcers over penis

-Fever with painless ulcers over penis

-Fever with whitish discharge in penis

-Fever with pain around the Umbilicus

-Fever with pain in the abdomen during deep inspiration

-Fever with over flank area of abdomen

-Fever with back pain

-Fever with discharging sinuses in the groin

It's Time To See The DOCTOR

-Fever with generalized tiredness

-Fever with loss of sleep

-Fever with headache and disorientation

-Fever with psychiatric complaints

-Fever with Petechial spots over the skin (purple or red spots in the skin)

-Fever with red spots over the abdomen and all over the body

-Fever present for every other day

-Fever present for every second day

-Fever present for every third day

-Fever present for more than 3 days

-Fever present for more than one week

-Fever present for more the one month

-Fever present for more than one month with diarrhea

-Fever present for more than one month and loss of body weight

-Fever with loss of weight more than 10% of body weight

-Fever with chronic cough with sputum

-Fever with chronic dry cough like barking

-Fever with generalized lymph node enlargement in the body

-Fever with white discharge from vagina in female

-Fever with toothache

-Fever with swelling of lips

-Fever with loss of expression in one side of face

-Fever with inability to close one eye

-Fever with loss of consciousness

-Fever with seizures

-Fever with weakness of limps

-Fever with altered behavior

-Fever with obscene behavior towards unknown women

-Fever with photophobia (fear to see the light)

-Fever with throat obstruction

-Fever with muscle spasm

-Fever with deviation of eye to one side and paralysis of extremities on the opposite side

-Fever with tongue deviation to one side

-Fever with paralysis of limbs

-Fever with abdomen pain that radiates to back

-Fever following outside food

-Fever following outside water drinking episode

-Fever following tick bite

-Fever following mountain climbing

-Fever following travel to foreign countries

-Fever following unprotected sexual intercourse

It's Time To See The DOCTOR

-Fever following eating meat and seafood and chicken

-Fever following handling of birds

-Fever following handling of animal products

-Fever following handling of animals

-Fever following agricultural work

-Fever following insect bite

-Fever following animal bite

-Fever following human bite

-Fever following biting of mothers nipple by infant

-Fever following baby's refusal to feed mothers milk from nipple

-Fever following injury

-Fever following inhalation of dust

-Fever following would infection

-Fever following abortion

-Fever following missed abortion

-Fever following swelling over the eyelids and inside of the eyelids

-Fever following headache

DR.K. Murugesan ,M.B.B.S.,

-Fever following self -injection of drugs by IV drug addicts

-Fever, vaginal discharge and lower abdomen pain

So ,if you have any of the complaints above consult your family physician and he would do appropriate tests and refer you to a Multispecialty hospital for further treatment.

2 HEAD ACHE

Whenever someone complaints of headache we must first find out the cause. For that you must first consult a doctor. There are many types of headaches. Tension type, Cluster type, Migraine, and brain tumor, Intra cerebral bleeding, bleeding around the brain to name a few causes. So if you have headache you should immediately consult a general physician and he would refer you to a multispecialty hospital for further management. There you would be consulted by a general physician, ENT doctor, eye doctor, Neuro physician and Neuro surgeon and vascular physician and they would work as a team and would order appropriate tests to find out the cause and give proper treatment.

If you have any of the following complaints you should consult your family physician as soon as possible.

-Headache with vomiting

-Headache with eye pain

-Headache with eye discharge

-Headache with inability to see light

-Headache aggravated by seeing light

-Headache with lacrimation

-Headache with giddiness

-Headache present on one side

-Headache present during the time of menses in women

-Headache with visual hallucination

-Headache with double vision

-Head ache on temporal region

-Headache over frontal region

-Headache in between eyes

-Headache when bending

-Headache more severe during night times

-Headache more severe during morning hours

-Headache followed by neck stiffness

-Most severe headache in my life ever

-Headache while speaking

-Headache during the time of stress

-Headache following head injury

-Headache followed by altered consciousness

-Headache followed by disorientation to time ,place, and person

-Headache followed by unconsciousness

-Headache followed by seizures

-Headache followed by nose bleeding

-Headache followed by nose block

-Headache followed by breathing difficulty

It's Time To See The DOCTOR

-Headache around the head like a band

-Headache with lacrimation and running nose

-Headache with eye pain

-Headache followed by weakness of extremities

-Headache followed by loss of speech

-Headache followed by loss of sensation in one side of body

-Minor head injury followed by over weeks to months of gradually increasing headache

-Headache followed by loss of vision

-Headache present during lying down and reduces while standing up

-Headache associated with aura like visual disturbances, photophobia

-Headache more severe in the morning

-Headache more severe in the night

-One sided headache

-Headache exacerbated during mensuration

-Headache around the eyes associated with lacrimation

-Sudden onset of severe headache

-Headache associated with neck stiffness and neurological deterioration

-Headache associated with dysphagia (difficulty in speech)

-Headache followed by mental changes

If you have Headache of any of the types above consult your family Physician and he/she would refer you to appropriate specialty doctors for further treatment .So don't ignore headache as simple headache always .

A brain tumor would usually present as headache of comes and goes nature and the headache would increase in severity depending upon the tumor growth and complications .Only after taking a CT scan or MRI scan we would be able to find out brain tumors. So as soon as you consult your doctor for headache he would be able to find out the correct diagnosis at the starting point of the disease and would be able to give you appropriate treatment to cure the disease.

3 VOMITING

Vomiting may be due to food poisoning or diseases in the stomach and intestines or due to generalized infection .So you must consult a general physician immediately if you have any of the following complaints

-Vomiting following food intake

-Vomiting following within hours of food intake

-Vomiting following 2-3 hours after food intake

-Vomiting following 1-2 days after food intake

-Vomiting followed by blood stained stools followed by epilepsy

-Vomiting with stomach pain and loose stools

Vomiting with regurgitation of food

-Vomiting of bile stained content

-Vomiting following alcohol drinking

-Vomiting of blood after alcohol drinking

-Vomiting followed by eating of egg, meat ,chicken, sea food,

-Vomiting with loose stools

-Vomiting with severe stomach pain

-Vomiting with giddiness

-Vomiting with chest pain followed by loss of consciousness

-Vomiting with loose stools and fever

- Self- induced vomiting after eating large meals in adolescent girls

-Vomiting of blood followed by cough

-Vomiting of blood in a patient with history of stomach ulcers

-Vomiting of blood in a patient with history of known chronic liver disease

-Vomiting of blood in a patient with history of known cancer

-Vomiting of blood in a patient with history of TB,HIV

-Vomiting in women of child bearing age

So if you have any of these symptoms immediately consult your family physician and he/she would refer you to a multispecialty hospital for further tests and the specialty doctors in a multispecialty hospital would work as a team and order appropriate test to find out the cause and give correct treatment.

4 LOOSE STOOLS

Loose stools may be due to acute gastroenteritis or may be due to some auto immune diseases like Ulcerative colitis or Crohn's disease. So you must consult a general physician and he/she would refer you to multispecialty hospital to find out the cause and give you proper treatment.

If you have any of the following complaints consult your family physician immediately.

-5-10 times of loose stools per day

-More than 10 times of loose stools per day

-Loose stools of rice water consistency

-Loose stools with stools mixed with blood

-Loose stools with stools mixed with worms

-Loose stools with generalized weakness

-Loose stools with fever

-Loose stools with giddiness while standing up

-Loose stools with dryness of mouth

-Loose stools with thirsty sensation

-Loose stools with reduced urine output

-Loose stools mixed with fat

-Loose stools mixed with mucus and blood

-Loose stools with stools floating on water

-Loose stools with foul smell

-Loose stools with dryness of skin

-Loose stools with loss of consciousness

-Loose stools with abdomen pain

-Loose stools with breathing difficulty

-Loose stools for more than a month

-Loose stools with loss of more than 10% of body weight

So , if you have any of these complaints above immediately consult your family physician and he would do appropriate examination and tests and refer you to a multispecialty hospital for admission and further management.

5 RESPIRATORY INFECTIONS

Running nose

A frequent complaint in pediatric population . The causes of running nose are the upper respiratory infections and climate changes. so it is better to consult a pediatrician regarding the complaint and follow his advice.

Sore throat

Sore throat is a most common complaint in pediatric and adult population . Sore throat is a sign of infection of the throat .Later it may lead to lower respiratory tract infection. It may lead to infection of larynx and trachea and may cause frequent dry cough . Most of the infections are harmless and Streptococcal infections will cause Rheumatic fever and IGA nephropathy. So you must consult your pediatrician to get proper advice.

Ear pain and Ear discharge

Ear pain and ear discharge are the most common complaints in children. In children immune system is not well developed and they are affected with dangerous bacterial species like pus forming staphylococcus aureus. So you must consult a pediatrician or general physician to get proper advice and treatment.

6 DISEASES IN CHILDREN

Children less than 1 year

children less than 1 year must be consulted by a Pediatrician or general physician with training in pediatric patients. Children are not small adults .there body functions and metabolism are not same as that of adults. So dose reduction of drugs according to their age is not effective. So children dose of drugs are calculated based upon body weight. So children less than 1 year must always be seen by a pediatrician or a general practitioner with training in Pediatric population. Children less than 1 year should be evaluated by a pediatrician for developmental milestones. Pediatrician would evaluate child's hearing ability , tone of muscles and child's ability to sit, stand and walk and speech development .So children less than one year must be evaluated by a pediatrician. Doctors will find out the causes and give their best treatment to cure the developmental defect.

Any child having sudden deep yellow or red discoloration of eyes should be brought to a pediatrician .

Discolored and hyper pigmented patches present over the body of a Newborn child. Should I consult the doctor?

Yes. You should see a pediatrician to find out the condition is benign or malignant .Some of the conditions would be entirely normal occurrence and some of the conditions would be dangerous. So it is better to see a pediatrician to get your doubts clarified.

Night blindness

You should immediately rush your child to your family physician, since it may be a reversible cause of blindness. Vitamin A deficiency is a common vitamin deficiency in childhood and it is reversible with supplementation of vitamin A . As soon you have seen a Pediatrician he/she would give treatment and give advice regarding how to prevent Vitamin A deficiency in future.

Vitamin D deficiency

Child's skull is flexible like a ball . Child's legs are bending forward and sideways while standing. It may be a sign of Vitamin D deficiency . Consult a pediatrician or general physician to get advice and treatment.

Vitamin C deficiency

There is easy bruising over the legs and extremities and minor bleeding occurs around the hair follicles and itching and minor bleeding occurs while scratching near thighs .Gum bleeding occurs while brushing teeth. This condition should be consulted with your family physician and he/she would order appropriate tests and give your proper treatment.

My child is having epilepsy whenever she gets fever. Is it an emergency?

Children less than 5 years will have epilepsy whenever the

temperature rises more than 100 degree Fahrenheit . It is called febrile seizures .Even though majority of them are harmless ,some of them would have some serious brain pathology. So you must immediately consult your family physician or Pediatrician and follow their advice and give proper treatment to your children.

My child is crying frequently . Should I see the doctor?

Infant are not able to tell you what problems they are having and it is an indication of underlying painful conditions .The child may be having severe Ear ache, Severe abdomen pain. So rush the child immediately to a Pediatrician and follow his or her advice.

My child is overactive. Should I see the doctor?

It is good to see a child active .Over activeness needs to be consulted with your family physician. Your Pediatrician would do appropriate tests and give your child proper treatment.

Consult your family physician if your child has the following complaints:

-A child present with short stature and swelling of abdomen, face and lower extremities

-A child present with short stature , low weight, reduced muscle mass

- High spiking fever for 5 or more days and rash , Conjunctivitis , strawberry appearing tongue , peeling of skin of extremities

-Fever for five days and disappearance of fever on fifth day and appearance of rash

-Recurrent diarrhea in children, failure to thrive and lymphadenopathy

-Small baby at birth, Low Platelet count , Jaundice, Small Head

-Anemia , swelling of limps face and abdomen in a just born child

-Watery diarrhea followed by blood streaked stools ,fever, abdomen pain and tiredness

-watery diarrhea followed by lower extremity weakness in two to three weeks after diarrhea

-Cat bite followed by fever, malaise, headache, anorexia

-Chronic diarrhea and failure to thrive

-Acute diarrhea and fever, tiredness, low grade fever, abdomen pain, nausea, foul smelling stools and abdomen distention

-Diarrhea, irritability, vomiting, loss of appetite, failure to thrive

-Night time bedwetting after being dry for at least 6 months

-Recurrent infection with pus forming organisms

-Development of rash in a previously healthy child over extensor surface of lower extremities and joint pain and abdomen pain

-Intermittent fever associated with salmon rash and the rash migrates to nearby areas

-Children with high spiking fevers associated with joint pain

-Children with high spiking fevers associated with joint pain and swelling

-Pain in scrotum associated with swelling in adolescent boys

7 DISEASES IN ADULT POPULATION

My husband will tell jokes while eating food and use to laugh. Is it normal?

Laughing is not advisable while eating food .It may lead to some serious conditions like chocking of food in the larynx . Kindly consult your family physician and follow his advice. He/she would be able to clarify your doubts and give proper advice.

My husband eats food while lying in the bed . Should I see the doctor?

Food must always be eaten by upright position. Food should not be eaten by lying down. It may lead to aspiration and breathing difficulties. Consult your doctor to get complete details and follow advice regarding this.

A normal man whose speech is good and suddenly deteriorates and he babbles while speaking .Should I see a doctor immediately?

Yes. It is a medical emergency. You should immediately rush him to a multispecialty hospital since it may be a stroke in the brain . Doctors would check his blood pressure and take a CT scan or MRI scan to find out the cause and give treatment . Your duty was to rush him immediately to a Multispecialty hospital and other things doctors would take care .

I do not have any complaints .Should I see the doctor?

Even though you do not have any complaints , depending upon your age there are health Check Ups .So consult your family doctor and He/she would guide you regarding the available health Check Up options and would refer you to a multispecialty hospital.

If you have Hypertension your family physician would ask you to come for regular blood pressure Check Up and would refer you to appropriate specialty doctors for further treatment

If you have Diabetes Mellitus your family physician would ask you to come for frequent blood sugar Check Up and refer you to a Diabetalogist and appropriate specialty doctors for further treatment

If you have chest pain you must consult your family physician and a cardiologist for regular follow up and treatments. For chest pain special investigations should be done to find any immediate treatment options. Your cardiologist will guide you correctly regarding the same. So you would rush to a multispecialty hospital to see a cardiologist if you were to have a chest pain.

Palpitation

Palpitation may be because of anxiety. We cannot ignore other causes like Anemia, Unknown gastrointestinal bleeding and hyperthyroidism. So you must see the general physician and he/she would refer you to a multispecialty hospital for further treatment.

Unintentional weight loss

You must see the doctor to find out the cause. Unintentional recent weight loss may be due to Hyperthyroid , TB to name a few diseases. So you should consult your family physician for complete Check Up and he/she would refer you to a multispecialty hospital for further treatment.

Jaundice

Dark yellowish discoloration of urine and Yellowish discoloration of conjunctiva in eyes. The causes of jaundice are many. Infective causes are Hepatitis, Malaria, Enteric fever, Dengue fever, Leptospirosis and Auto immune causes like primary biliary cirrhosis , liver cancer, Pancreatic cancer , bile duct calculi to name a few diseases . So whenever a jaundice occurs in adult population , she or he must see a general physician immediately and based on his advice you would see specialist doctors and get admitted in a multispecialty hospital and do all tests to find out the cause and get proper treatment. So the cause must be found out in jaundice to get correct treatment. So never ignore jaundice as there may be some serious underlying causes.

If jaundice occurs in newborn infant in the first week of life , there are both harmless and harmful conditions and a Neonatologist should be consulted as soon as possible. If the delivery occurred in the hospital , the doctors in the hospital would explain you about the condition of the child and they would give proper treatment.

Tremors of hands

Some of the people may have tremors of hand and feet since childhood and it may be essential tremor. Tremor may occur during the time of anxiety also. Some of the tremors occur because of a lesion in the brain and are harmful and needs to be treated.

So if you come to know that you have any kind of tremor the first thing is to see a general physician and he/she would refer you to a multispecialty hospital to see neurologist and appropriate specialist doctors to get proper treatment.

Muscles and Joints

-If there is progressive swelling of calf and unable to walk in young age

- If there was swelling in big toe associated with pain with no history of injury

-If there was swelling of wrists and ankles

-If there was swelling of fingers and toes

-If there was pain in all joints in the early hours of waking and disappears as the day progresses

-If there was no pain in the joints during early hours of waking and pain increases as the day progresses

-If there was knee pain associated with vision problems

-If there was joint pain and wounds and ulcers over the scrotum

-If there was joint pain associated with fever

-If there was joint pain in the shoulders and pelvis and unable to lift the hands above head and unable to sit without pain

-If joint pain associated with urethral discharge

-If there is low back pain and hip pain or neck pain which increases during rest

-If joint pain associated with skin changes and nail changes

-If join pain associated with fever

It's time to see your family physician and he/she would refer you to a multispecialty hospital where all specialty doctors would be available and work as a team to find out the cause and give you correct treatment.

Epilepsy

Sudden involuntary flexion and extension of all four limbs followed by Unconsciousness and tongue biting and involuntary urination and consciousness slowly regained and immediately after the patient presents with confusion and then becomes normal

Sudden involuntary flexion and Extension of one limb without loss of consciousness

Sudden involuntary flexion and extension of one limb with loss of consciousness

Sudden unresponsiveness for 5-10 sec by starring and return to normal behavior as if nothing had occurred

Seizures in a child less than 6 months with positive family history of seizures

Seizures occurring in a child less than 5 years during the time of fever

If anything above happens consult your family physician and he would refer you to a multispecialty hospital for further investigations and proper treatment.

Vertigo

-Transient and frequent vertigo

-Vertigo associated with nausea and vomiting

-Vertigo associated with hearing disturbances and hearing loss

-Vertigo associated with change in head position

So, It's time to see your family physician and he would refer you to a multispecialty hospital for further investigations and management.

Syncope

-Sudden loss of consciousness for less than 30 sec and immediate return to consciousness

-Syncope associated with any precipitating events like standing for a long time ,hearing sounds, seeing blood, seeing heights

You should consult your family physician and he would refer you to a neurologist, vascular surgeon and general physician or ENT surgeon and neurologist and cardiologist in a multispecialty hospital and they would work as a team and find out the cause by ordering appropriate investigations and would give you proper treatment.

Weakness

-Inability to lift the eyelids

-Double vision as the day progresses

-Inability to lift arms above shoulders

-Normal in the morning and progressive weakness in the evening

-Progressive chronic weakness of arms, shoulder and limbs over months

-Progressive ascending weakness starting in the lower limbs and extending to abdomen and shoulders

-Loss of sensation in one part of the body

-Relapsing and remitting type of eye pain

If you have any of these complaints you must consult your family physician and he would refer you to a multispecialty hospital for further treatment

Dementia

-Loss of memory to recent events

-Loss of memory to new events

-progressive loss of memory leading to forgetfulness of daily routine activities

-Loss of memory to known subjects

-Like not able to name pen as pen ,rose as rose and naming them as this and that

-Sudden deterioration of memory and inappropriate behavior over opposite sex

-Suddenly become inappropriate person and making sexual comments to unknown people

-Sudden loss of all memories with associated history of hypertension and diabetes

These complaints of memory loss should be investigated in a multispecialty hospital and they would do appropriate tests to find out the cause and treat accordingly

Movements

-Sudden appearance of involuntary dance like purposeless movements

-Tremors at rest

-Inability to stand up from sitting position

-Inability to walk straight

-Swaying to one side while walking

-Tendency to fall while walking

-Abnormal walking pattern

-Involuntary nodding of head

These should be evaluated by a neurologist in a multispecialty hospital. They would do appropriate investigations to find out the cause and would give appropriate treatment.

Eye pain

-Eye pain associated with progressive dimness of vision

-Eye pain associated with impaired adaptation to darkness

-sudden appearance of visual bloaters

-sudden loss of vision

These complaints should be evaluated by an eye doctor and he would refer you to a multispecialty hospital for further management.

Abdomen pain

-Sudden abdomen pain around the umbilicus , all over the abdomen, upper abdomen, flanks and epigastrium,

-Abdomen pain on and off for more than one month

-Abdomen pain relieved by eating food

-Abdomen pain starts after eating food

-Abdomen pain radiates to back

If you have any of these complaints you must consult your family physician and he/she would refer you to a gastroenterologist and he would refer you to a multispecialty hospital for further tests and treatment.

8 BIRTH DEFECTS IN CHILDREN

-Upward deviation of eyes

-Downward deviation of eyes

-Low set ears

-Big ears

-Small mouth

-Small eyes

-Big eyes

-Eye in the forehead near midline

-Midline facial clefts

-Rocker bottom feet

-More than 5 digits in hands and feet

-Fused digits in hands and feet

-Small stature

It's Time To See The DOCTOR

-Webbed neck

-Increased distance between nipples

-Swelling of feet

-Small head

-Big head

-Complete absence of speech

-Poor feeding

-Micro penis

-Fused vagina

-Flaccid limbs

-Decreased hearing

-Bloody urine

-Frothy urine

-Presence of more than five fingers or toes

-Fusing of two or more fingers or toes

-Cleft lip

-Cleft palate

-Curvature of penis downward

-Urethral opening on undersurface of penis

-Odor of maple syrup in urine and sweat

-Mental retardation

-Blind and deaf by one year of age

-Stiff joints

-Loose joints

-Thin extremities

-Big tongue

-Small chin

-Big abdomen

-Abdomen swelling

-Child with self- injurious behavior

-Abnormal facial features

-short neck

-low hairline

-limited neck motion

-twisted neck

-Prominent calf muscles

-tall stature

-long and thin extremities

-Hyper extensibility of joints

-double head

-conjoined twins

It's Time To See The DOCTOR

-Child with coarse facial features

-Child with restricted joint movements

-Child with hands looking like waiter's tip

-Child with hands looking like claw hand

-Child with shoulder bones looking like wings of birds

-Self- mutilation and aggressive behaviour in a child

-Orange colored crystals in diaper of child

-Difficulty with movement in a child

-Frequent infection in a child

-Freckle like increased pigmentation and mottled appearing pigmentation of skin in a child

-Child with birdlike facial appearance, Large ears, small head ,thin nose, short stature, long extremities

-Child present with scaly skin (fish skin)

-Pallor, small red color spots over the skin and bruises

-Child present with butterfly like facial rash

-Child with disproportionally aged like appearance

-Allery to x-rays, dull and relaxed facial appearance, aged looking skin

-Large infant with large tongue and small head

-Stroke in a child

-Unequal leg length and asymmetry of thigh skin creases

-Severe joint contractures

-Short and broad fingers

-Unequal leg length and asymmetry of thigh skin creases

-Severe joint contractures

-Short and broad fingers

-Extra digits in hands and feet

-Bent fingers

-Curvature of the finger

-Absent thumb

-Short and bowed forearm

-One lower extremity shorter than the other

-One thigh shorter than other thigh

-One foot shorter than the other and it lies at the level opposite to other knee

-Anterior bowing of leg

-Lateral bowing of leg

-Hyperextension of leg

-Hyperextension of knee joint

-Hyperextension of ankle joint

-Bending of leg in children

-Abnormal walking pattern in children and adults

-Hammer like deformity of toes

-Mallet like deformity of toes

-Claw like deformity of toes

-Loss of normal arch of foot

-Flat foot

-In growing toe nail in thumb

-Overlapping of 5th toe over other toes

-Curly toes

-One or more large digits in hands and feet

So , if any of these abnormal appearance occurs in newborn child you should immediately consult a pediatrician in a multispecialty hospital. There may be defects in many organ systems in the body or they be harmless. These things could not be told by external examination alone. These newborn infants must be examined by various specialty doctors to find out the exact defects inside the body.

A cardiologist should be consulted to find out heart defects.

An Endocrinologist must be consulted to find defects in secretory and endocrine glands.

A Neurologist must be consulted to find out defects in the brain.

An orthopedician must be consulted to find out defects in the bones.

An oncologist must be consulted to find out the possibility of cancer in future.

A cardio thoracic surgeon must be consulted to find out any defects in lungs and heart.

A gastroenterologist must be consulted to find out defects in the stomach and intestines.

A general surgeon must be consulted to find out congenital hernias.

An ophthalmologist must be consulted to find out defects in the eyes

An ENT surgeon must be consulted to find out defects in the ear, nose and throat

A physiotherapist must be consulted to find out what kind of rehabilitation therapy needed.

So if you rush to a multispecialty hospital , all specialty doctors would be available .They would all work as a team and find out defects and would give you best appropriate treatment to have a near normal life.

9 INFECTIONS IN NEWBORN CHILD

-All newborn infants should be seen by a pediatrician regarding vaccination schedule.

-Any infant with multiple injury may be abused by their parents.

-Excessive bleeding from circumcision site

-Frequent respiratory infection

-Urinary tract infections

-Gastro intestinal infections

-Fever with poor feeding

-Fever high grade with rashes

-Fever with breathing difficulties

-Fever associated with vomiting, nausea, abdomen pain, headache seizures, loose stools, generalized malaise and poor feeding

-Fever with cough, wheezing and seizures

-Excessive spitting up in the first week of life

-Sudden appearance of high pitched cry

-Vomiting after feeding and progressive in nature after one month of age

-Bile stained vomiting on the first week of life

-Abdomen pain ,bile stained vomiting and currant jelly stool at 3 months to 5 years of age

-Intermittent painless anal bleeding

-Abdomen pain in children around umbilicus

-Cough with running nose

-Dry cough or productive cough

-Cough followed by drooling of saliva5

-Cough followed by sputum mixed with blood

-Cough followed by wheezing

-Cough and fever

-Cough and sore throat

-Cough followed by breathing difficulty

-Pain with swallowing

-Refusal to swallow due to pain

-High fever with difficulty swallowing

- Increased drooling in first week of age and choking and cough and cyanosis on attempted feeding

-Nose bleeding

-Breathing difficulty that improves on crying , breathing difficulty during feeding

-Limp and unable to bear weight

-Multiple fractures after minor injury

-Hereditary spherocytosis, elliptocytosis, Sickle cell anemia and Thalassemia and G6PD deficiency are red blood cell diseases

-Chediak-Higashi syndrome and chronic granulomatous diseases arise from abnormal neutrophil function.

So , It's time to see the pediatric doctor for complete examination and further treatment . He/she would refer the child to a multispecialty children's hospital for appropriate test and further treatment.

10 DISORDERS OF CHILD DEVELOPMENT

-Disobedient child

-Aggressive behavior with people and animal

-Hyperactive child

-Inattentive child

-Involuntary frequent blinking of eyes

-Frequency use of obscene words

-Exact repetition of words

-Abnormal movement of body parts

-Loss of interest in activities

-Depressed mood

-Suicide attempt

-Interest in wearing cloths of opposite sex

 -Interest in behavior of opposite sex

- Thinking in his/her mind the he/she belongs to opposite sex

-Frequent dieting and losing weight and refusing to feed for fear of gaining weight

-Frequent feeding of large meals and followed by self- induced vomiting

- Excessive concern about large nose and small muscles

These symptoms must be consulted with your family physician and pediatrician and they would refer the child to appropriate consultants for further tests and appropriate diagnosis and treatment.

11 ENDOCRINE GLAND DISEASES

-Dark pigmentation on inside of the mouth

-Prominent ridges above the eyes and exaggerated wrinkles and thickened facial appearance, plump lips and exaggerated lower jaw

-Men appearing like well-built rugby player or boxer with rough facial appearance

-Prominent frontal bones

-Thickened skin with indistinct features

-Large and round face

-Distinct contours pf nose

-Large nose and facial features

-Prominent muscular contours in face

-Jaw gradually increases in size and becomes large

-Thick wide and large tongue

-Large nose and thick supra orbital ridges

-Disproportionately large nose

-Prominent lower jaw

-Large fleshy lips

-Large square tongue

-Thickened bulky tongue

-Over biting of lower teeth

-Large square feet

-Rounding of the face

-Facial plethora

-Moon face with obesity

-Hirsutism with facial flushing

-Central opacity with purple stretch marks

-Thin skin with underlying visible veins

-Paper like thin skin

-Needing a prop to stand up

-Lid retraction and buried eyelids

-Pretibial myxedema

-Clubbing of fingers

-Convex nails with swelling around nails

-Detachment of nail from nail bed

-Loss of weight despite increased dietary intake

-Heat intolerance , irritability, restlessness, palpitations,

-Diarrhea, extreme tiredness

-Hands are warm and moist

-Cold and sweaty hands in simple anxiety

-Fine tremor on outstretched hands

-Mentally and physically slow

-Obese with non-pitting edema

-Dry inelastic and cold skin

-Thick and croaky voice

-Progressive darkening of skin

-Tiredness, dizziness, anorexia, weight loss, cramps, nausea, vomiting and depression

-Pigmentation overs gums and buccal mucosa

-Loss of pubic hair in females

-Hyperpigmentation of fingers

-Deep palmar creases

Kindly consult your family physician if you find any of these symptoms above to get proper advice and treatment.

12 CONSULTATION OF DOCTOR FOLLOWING INJURY

-Brief loss of consciousness following head injury

 -Patient asks same question again and again after head injury

-Consciousness followed by loss of consciousness after head injury

-Avoid unnecessary manipulation of neck following head injury

-Extremely weak hand shake following car accident involving sudden stoppage of the car during heavy speed where the passenger's upper body would swing like a whiplash

-Breathing difficulty following injury to chest with sharp objects

-Chest injury followed by palpitation

-Any abdomen injury by blunt or sharp objects

-Penetrating injury of abdomen by sharp objects

-Penetrating injury of chest by sharp or blunt objects

-Dizziness, Diplopia, Dysphagia and Vertical spontaneous movement of one or both eyes following injury to head

   If you find any of these symptoms after injury kindly consult your family physician and he would refer you to the proper consultant doctor for further management.

13 BONE DISEASES

-Progressive enlargement of head followed by headache , Progressive bowing of limbs and Sudden deafness

-Muscular over development in children

-Ask a person To perform hand shake and observe . If he finds difficult in releasing grasp he must be referred to a neurologist for further investigations and management.

-Painless enlargement of shoulder joint

-Painless enlargement of ankle joint

-Painless enlargement of knee joint

-Painless enlargement of any joint in the body

-Loss of sensation in foot

-Loss of sensation in any part of the body.

-Loss of sensation to touch and temperature.

- Fever, joint pain followed by restriction of joint movements

-Joint pain , swelling followed by restriction of movement and refusal to walk or stand in children

-Opening in the skin and drainage of pus through the opening

-Sudden onset of swelling and pain in a joint followed by fever and malaise and inability to walk due to pain

-History of injury followed by swelling of joint and joint pain

-Loss of gluteal fold in one buttock

-Pain over bone, mass over bone, abnormal shape of bone, fracture of bone without injury, pain in the bone present continuously at rest, pain present in night times, pain increases slightly during walk

-Fracture of bone following minor injury

-Palpable mass in abdomen

-Painless mass over back, thorax, abdomen and neck

-Confusion and appearance of blood spots over skin after bone surgery

-Wrist drop following fracture

-Foot drop following fracture

-Prolonged compression of limp as in alcoholic patients

-If child's shirt hangs asymmetrically even after proper wearing

-Joint pain at extremes of motion and loss of both active and passive motion

-Popping sound and sharp pain over joint or muscle following lifting of weight

-Jobs involving repetitive workload on the elbow

-If you are an active tennis player

and if you have elbow pain following opening of door and

turning a screw driver you should see the doctor

-If you are a golf player and have elbow pain

-Pain in forearm aggravated by lifting weight

-Pain in elbow following throwing activity in athletes

-Catching and giving way of elbow

-Mild limitation of elbow extension and abnormal swelling at elbow without prior history of injury

-Swan neck deformity of fingers

-Slow onset of wrist pain that increase with activity

-Unable to extend one or more fingers and pain on passive extension

-Pain during repetitive thumb movement

-Dimpling and puckering of skin in palm of hands

-palpable nodule in palm of hands

-Firm rubbery swelling over wrist

-Pain and swelling of digits

-Swelling and pain of tip of fingers

Kindly consult your family physician immediately to get proper advice and he would refer you to a specialty doctor for further management.

14 SKIN DISEASES

-Swelling of lips after using latex gloves

-Swelling of lips after touching balloon

-Frequent hand washing with detergent soap followed by lesions over fingers and finger tips

-Itching of hands following exposure of detergents and irritants

-Skin lesions following hot showers

-Cracked porcelain like lesions

- Itching over whole body in a patient with known history of asthma

-Itching over whole body on and off from childhood

-Itching of hands following use of juice from citrus fruits and use of soaps

-Skin irritation following exposure of acids, alkalis, antiseptics, waterless hand cleansers, hand soap, wet cement, dish detergents, shampoo, fruit acids , vinegar, turpentine, gasoline, benzene and kerosene

-Allergy following exposure to poison ivy, oak, sumac fragrances , preservatives, topical antibiotics

-Itching following wearing of Jewelry ,belt buckles, fingernail polish and hair products

-Itching following wearing of gloves, ear ring, Shoes, underclothing

-Itchy rash with coin shaped lesions on skin

-Itchy or painful blisters on palms and soles

-Itchy areas of skin with interruption of sleep

-Salmon colored plaques and silvery scales

-Itching followed by joint pain and swelling in hands and feet

-Rashes with white scales

-Rashes with pus formation

-Nail pitting and nail plate separation associated with joint pain

-Dry and itchy scalp

-Loose white flakes on scalp

-Respiratory infection followed by itchy skin lesions

-Single big itchy rash followed by small multiple rashes over body

-Itching and red bumps

-Nail plate thickening

-Black dots on skin

-Itching of scalp and hair loss

-Itching of scalp without hair loss

-Dandruff over the scalp

-Hair loss with black spots

-Hair loss with lymph node enlargement in nape of neck

Kindly consult your family physician for further referral to a skin doctor and proper consultants and further management.

15 DISEASES IN WOMEN

-Bleeding or spotting from vagina after sexual intercourse in women of Child bearing age

-Bleeding or spotting from vagina after sexual intercourse in women after menopause

-Bleeding or spotting after sexual intercourse may be normal during the first sexual intercourse or sometimes after

-Bleeding from vagina during the time of menses is normal.

-Heavy flow of bleeding during the time of menses may be abnormal

-Heavy Bleeding from vagina and pain abdomen during menses may be abnormal

-Scant vaginal bleeding during the time of menses may be abnormal

-Vaginal bleeding associated with clotted blood may be abnormal during the time of menses

-Menses present for only one day in a month may be abnormal

-Vaginal bleeding present for more than one week during menses may be abnormal

-Vaginal bleeding occurring at irregular intervals may be abnormal

-The gap between two menstrual cycles more than 45 day may be abnormal

-Two menses occurring in one month may be abnormal

-Menses occurring once every two months may be abnormal

-Menses occurring once every 3 months or longer may be abnormal

 If you find any of these complaints kindly consult your gynecology doctor for further management.

16 SCREENING FOR MULTIPLE DISEASES

-Family history of mental retardation

 -Testicular development only after puberty

-Pregnancy at an older age woman and delivery of a child with hearing loss and heart problems

-Girl with short stature, Webbed neck , low hairline and wide spaced nipples

-Rashes in the first week of life

-Hard stools , pain with defecation, failure to pass three stools per week , irritability, abdomen pain

-History of breast cancer in the family

-History of colon cancer in the family

-History of heart disease in the family

-History of hypertension in the family

-History of diabetes in the family

-History cancer in multiple organs in the family

ABOUT THE AUTHOR

The author of this book is DR .K. Murugesan . He is a doctor . He has finished M.B.B.S., and Has ten years of clinical experience In general medicine . He studied MBBS in GOVT KILPAUK MEDICAL COLLEGE ,Chennai, India. He studied school in GOVERNMENT HIGH SCHOOL,VELLANKOIL and KAMBAN KALVI NILAIYAM MATRICULATION HR.SEC.SCHOOL in Gobichettipalayam , Tamil Nadu . He is now working as a medical officer in VIJAYA HEALTH CENTRE , Vadapalani, Chennai and DOCTOR MURUGESAN CLINIC, Saligramam ,Chennai , INDIA .

DR.K. Murugesan ,M.B.B.S.,

It's Time To See The DOCTOR

www.ingramcontent.com/pod-product-compliance
Lightning Source LLC
Chambersburg PA
CBHW071726170526
45165CB00005B/2168